The Best Autoimmune Protocol Diet for Beginners

Nourishing Recipes for Breakfast, Lunch, and Dinner

By Ashley Johnson

Contents

Introduction

Embracing the Autoimmune Protocol Diet

The journey to health and well-being often begins with what we choose to nourish our bodies with. The Autoimmune Protocol (AIP) diet is a transformative approach designed to support those battling autoimmune diseases by reducing inflammation, healing the gut, and ultimately, promoting overall wellness. Rooted in the belief that food is medicine, the AIP diet eliminates potentially inflammatory foods and focuses on nutrient-dense, whole foods that provide essential vitamins and minerals. By removing triggers and introducing healing foods, the AIP diet helps individuals regain control over their health, one meal at a time.

Understanding the Foundations

The foundation of the AIP diet lies in its strict elimination phase, where common allergens and inflammatory foods such as grains, dairy, legumes, nightshades, and processed foods are removed from the diet. This phase, though challenging, is crucial for identifying food sensitivities and allowing the body to begin the healing process. Following this, the reintroduction phase allows for the careful and systematic reintroduction of eliminated foods to determine which ones may trigger symptoms. This approach not only helps in managing autoimmune conditions but also fosters a deeper understanding of one's body and its unique needs.

A Culinary Adventure

Embarking on the AIP diet does not mean sacrificing flavor or variety. In fact, it opens the door to a world of culinary creativity. This cookbook is your guide to nourishing your body with delicious and wholesome meals that adhere to the AIP guidelines. From hearty breakfasts that kickstart your day to satisfying lunches and dinners that leave you feeling nourished and energized, every recipe is crafted to support your health journey. The recipes within these pages are not only AIP-compliant but also easy to prepare, making your transition to this lifestyle as seamless as possible.

Your Path to Wellness

In "The Autoimmune Protocol Diet for Beginners: Nourishing Recipes for Breakfast, Lunch, and Dinner," you will find a collection of recipes designed to make the AIP diet enjoyable and sustainable. Each recipe is accompanied by tips and insights to help you make the most of your culinary experience. Whether you are new to the AIP diet or seeking fresh inspiration, this cookbook aims to empower you with the knowledge and tools needed to take charge of your health. As you explore these nourishing recipes, you will discover that healing through food is not only possible but also deliciously rewarding.

Welcome to a new chapter of your health journey, where each meal is a step towards a healthier, happier you.

The Importance of Breakfast

Breakfast is often called the most important meal of the day, and for good reason. It sets the tone for your energy levels and mood, providing the nutrients your body needs to start the day strong. In the context of the AIP diet, breakfast takes on even greater significance. This cookbook offers a variety of breakfast recipes that are not only AIP-compliant but also satisfying and delicious. From nutrient-packed smoothie bowls to hearty egg-free scrambles and comforting breakfast hashes, these recipes will help you kickstart your day with the right balance of protein, healthy fats, and fiber.

Nourishing Lunches

Lunchtime is an opportunity to refuel and recharge, especially when following the AIP diet. Our selection of lunch recipes is designed to keep you satiated and energized throughout the afternoon. You'll find an array of salads bursting with fresh, vibrant vegetables, protein-rich main dishes featuring fish and lean meats, and comforting soups and stews that are perfect for any season. Each recipe is crafted to be nutrient-dense and easy to prepare, ensuring that you can enjoy a wholesome, AIP-friendly meal even on your busiest days.

Satisfying Dinners

Dinner on the AIP diet is all about winding down with a nourishing, comforting meal that supports your body's healing process. This cookbook offers a variety of dinner recipes that are both satisfying and compliant with AIP guidelines. From flavorful roasted meats and fish to inventive vegetable dishes and hearty one-pot meals, these recipes are designed to be both simple and delicious. Whether you're cooking for yourself or sharing a meal with family and friends, these dinners will become staples in your weekly meal plan, making it easy to stick to your AIP journey.

Your AIP Kitchen Essentials

Transitioning to the AIP diet may seem daunting at first, but with the right tools and ingredients, it becomes much more manageable. This cookbook includes a comprehensive guide to stocking your AIP pantry, highlighting essential ingredients that will make your cooking experience smoother and more enjoyable. From coconut aminos and bone broth to a variety of herbs and spices that add depth and flavor without causing inflammation, this section ensures you have everything you need at your fingertips. Additionally, tips on meal prep and kitchen organization will help you save time and stay on track with your health goals.

In conclusion, "The Autoimmune Protocol Diet for Beginners: Nourishing Recipes for Breakfast, Lunch, and Dinner" is more than just a cookbook—it's a guide to reclaiming your health through the power of food. By embracing the principles of the AIP diet and incorporating these delicious, nutrient-dense recipes into your daily routine, you'll be well on your way to achieving a healthier, more vibrant life. Here's to your journey towards wellness, one nourishing meal at a time.

Embracing the Journey

As you embark on this journey, remember that the AIP diet is not just a temporary fix, but a long-term commitment to better health. The recipes in this cookbook are designed to be flexible and adaptable to your personal taste and lifestyle. Embracing the AIP diet means being open to exploring new ingredients and cooking techniques, and finding joy in nourishing your body with wholesome foods. It is a journey of discovery and empowerment, where you take control of your health and well-being one meal at a time.

Community and Support

One of the most important aspects of the AIP journey is finding a community of like-minded individuals who understand and support your goals. Whether through online forums, local support groups, or social media, connecting with others who are also following the AIP diet can provide invaluable support and motivation. Sharing recipes, tips, and experiences with others can help you stay on track and make the journey more enjoyable. Remember, you are not alone in this; there is a vibrant and supportive community ready to cheer you on.

Adapting to Your Needs

Every individual's journey on the AIP diet is unique. What works for one person may not work for another, and that's perfectly okay. This cookbook encourages you to listen to your body and make adjustments as needed. Pay attention to how different foods make you feel, and don't be afraid to experiment with substitutions and modifications to suit your preferences and dietary needs. The goal is to create a sustainable and enjoyable way of eating that supports your health and well-being in the long term.

Celebrating Progress

Finally, it's important to celebrate your progress along the way. The AIP diet can be challenging, but every step you take towards better health is a victory. Celebrate the small wins, whether it's discovering a new favorite recipe, feeling more energized, or noticing improvements in your symptoms. Keep a journal to track your journey, noting the positive changes and milestones you achieve. Remember, the AIP diet is a marathon, not a sprint, and every positive change you make is a step towards a healthier, happier you.

In closing, "The Autoimmune Protocol Diet for Beginners: Nourishing Recipes for Breakfast, Lunch, and Dinner" is your companion in this transformative journey. With its wealth of delicious, nutrient-dense recipes and practical tips, this cookbook aims to make the AIP diet accessible and enjoyable for everyone. By embracing the principles of the AIP diet and committing to nourishing your body with whole, healing foods, you are taking a powerful step towards reclaiming your health. Here's to your journey towards wellness—one nourishing meal at a time.

Fun Facts About the AIP Diet

1. Ancient Healing Wisdom

The AIP diet draws inspiration from ancestral diets and traditional healing practices. Many of the foods recommended in the AIP diet, such as bone broth and fermented vegetables, have been used for centuries in various cultures to promote health and longevity.

This diet reconnects us with time-tested wisdom about the healing power of food.

2. Gut Health Revolution

One of the primary goals of the AIP diet is to heal the gut. Did you know that the gut is often referred to as the "second brain"? It contains its own nervous system and produces many of the same neurotransmitters found in the brain, such as serotonin. By healing your gut, you can positively impact your mood, cognitive function, and overall well-being.

3. Hidden Food Sensitivities

The elimination phase of the AIP diet is a powerful tool for uncovering hidden food sensitivities. Many people are surprised to learn that foods they considered healthy, like tomatoes or eggs, can trigger inflammation in their bodies. Identifying and removing these triggers can lead to significant improvements in health and symptom management.

4. Nutrient Density

The AIP diet emphasizes nutrient-dense foods, meaning foods that are rich in vitamins, minerals, and other essential nutrients relative to their calorie content. Organ meats, seafood, and leafy greens are some of the most nutrient-dense foods on the planet, and they play a starring role in the AIP diet. This focus on nutrient density helps ensure that your body gets everything it needs to heal and thrive.

5. Creative Cooking

Following the AIP diet can be a fun and creative culinary adventure. With many common ingredients off the table, you'll have the opportunity to experiment with new foods and cooking techniques. You might discover a love for spiralized vegetables, cauliflower rice, or homemade coconut yogurt. This diet encourages you to think outside the box and find delicious new ways to enjoy your meals.

6. Mindful Eating

The AIP diet encourages a mindful approach to eating. By paying attention to how different foods affect your body, you become more attuned to your nutritional needs and how to best support your health. This mindfulness extends beyond the diet, fostering a deeper connection between you and your body's signals, leading to healthier choices in all areas of life.

7. Community and Connection

Many people find that the AIP diet brings them closer to their communities. Whether it's sharing recipes, participating in support groups, or attending AIP-friendly potlucks, the diet fosters a sense of connection and shared purpose. These relationships can provide essential support and encouragement throughout your healing journey.

8. Personalized Nutrition

The AIP diet is not a one-size-fits-all approach. It's designed to be personalized, allowing you to discover which foods work best for your unique body. This individualized approach to nutrition helps you create a diet that supports your specific health needs, making it more effective and sustainable in the long run.

9. Empowerment through Knowledge

By following the AIP diet, you'll gain a wealth of knowledge about nutrition, cooking, and your own body. This empowerment through knowledge is one of the most rewarding aspects of the diet. You'll become more confident in making dietary choices that support your health and well-being, and you'll have the tools to continue your healing journey for years to come.

10. A Path to Overall Wellness

While the primary focus of the AIP diet is on managing autoimmune conditions, many people experience broader health benefits as well. Improved energy levels, better sleep, clearer skin, and enhanced mental clarity are just a few of the positive changes reported by those following the AIP diet. This holistic approach to wellness underscores the profound impact that food can have on our overall health.

In conclusion, "The Autoimmune Protocol Diet for Beginners: Nourishing Recipes for Breakfast, Lunch, and Dinner" is more than just a collection of recipes—it's a guide to a healthier, more vibrant life. By embracing the AIP diet, you are taking an important step towards healing and wellness. Enjoy the journey, and remember to savor each nourishing meal along the way.

BREAKFAST

1. Sweet Potato Hash with Ground Turkey

Prep Time: 25 minutes

Ingredients:

- 2 medium sweet potatoes, peeled and diced
- 1 lb ground turkey
- 1 small onion, diced
- 1 red bell pepper, diced
- 2 tbsp coconut oil
- 1 tsp sea salt
- 1/2 tsp black pepper (optional for strict AIP)
- 1 tsp dried thyme

Instructions:

1. Heat coconut oil in a large skillet over medium heat.
2. Add diced sweet potatoes and cook until they start to soften (about 10 minutes).
3. Add the onion and bell pepper, cooking until the onion is translucent.
4. Add ground turkey, breaking it up with a spoon, and cook until browned.
5. Season with salt, pepper (if using), and thyme.
6. Serve hot.

Tip: You can make a large batch and reheat portions throughout the week.

Fun Fact: Sweet potatoes are rich in beta-carotene, which the body converts to vitamin A, important for immune health.

2. Apple-Cinnamon Breakfast Bowl

Prep Time: 10 minutes

Ingredients:

- 1 large apple, peeled, cored, and diced
- 1/4 cup unsweetened applesauce
- 1 tbsp coconut butter
- 1/2 tsp ground cinnamon
- 1 tbsp shredded coconut (optional)
- 1 tbsp pumpkin seeds (optional for strict AIP)

Instructions:

1. In a small saucepan, combine the apple, applesauce, and coconut butter.
2. Cook over medium heat until the apple is soft, about 5-7 minutes.
3. Stir in the cinnamon and cook for another minute.
4. Serve topped with shredded coconut and pumpkin seeds if using.

Tip: For a creamier texture, blend the cooked mixture before adding toppings.

Fun Fact: Apples are a great source of fiber, which is beneficial for gut health.

3. Plantain Pancakes

Prep Time: 20 minutes

Ingredients:

- 2 large green plantains, peeled and chopped

- 2 eggs (or 2 tbsp gelatin dissolved in 4 tbsp water for egg-free)
- 2 tbsp coconut flour
- 1 tsp baking soda
- 1/2 tsp sea salt
- Coconut oil for cooking

Instructions:

1. Blend plantains in a food processor until smooth.
2. Add eggs, coconut flour, baking soda, and salt, blending until well combined.
3. Heat coconut oil in a skillet over medium heat.
4. Pour batter to form small pancakes and cook until bubbles form on the surface. Flip and cook until golden brown.
5. Serve with fresh berries or a drizzle of honey.

Tip: Use ripe plantains for a sweeter pancake.

Fun Fact: Plantains are a staple in many tropical regions and are more starchy than bananas.

4. Avocado and Smoked Salmon Breakfast Bowl

Prep Time: 10 minutes

Ingredients:

- 1 ripe avocado, diced
- 3 oz smoked salmon
- 1 cup mixed greens
- 1 tbsp extra-virgin olive oil
- 1 tbsp lemon juice
- Sea salt to taste

Instructions:

1. Arrange mixed greens in a bowl.
2. Top with diced avocado and smoked salmon.
3. Drizzle with olive oil and lemon juice.
4. Season with sea salt and serve.

Tip: Use a variety of greens for different textures and flavors.

Fun Fact: Avocados are high in healthy fats and potassium, supporting heart health and electrolyte balance.

5. Coconut Yogurt Parfait

Prep Time: 15 minutes

Ingredients:

- 1 cup coconut yogurt
- 1/2 cup mixed berries
- 2 tbsp unsweetened shredded coconut
- 1 tbsp honey (optional)
- 1 tbsp chia seeds (optional)

Instructions:

1. Layer coconut yogurt and berries in a serving bowl.
2. Sprinkle with shredded coconut and chia seeds.
3. Drizzle with honey if desired.

Tip: Make your own coconut yogurt for a probiotic-rich breakfast.

Fun Fact: Chia seeds are packed with omega-3 fatty acids, which are anti-inflammatory and beneficial for brain health.

6. Butternut Squash and Bacon Egg Muffins

Prep Time: 30 minutes

Ingredients:

- 1 small butternut squash, peeled and diced
- 4 slices of bacon, chopped
- 6 eggs (or 6 tbsp gelatin dissolved in 12 tbsp water for egg-free)
- 1/2 tsp sea salt
- 1/4 tsp black pepper (optional for strict AIP)
- 1/2 tsp garlic powder

Instructions:

1. Preheat oven to 350°F (175°C) and grease a muffin tin.
2. Cook bacon in a skillet until crispy, then set aside.
3. In the same skillet, cook the butternut squash until tender.
4. In a bowl, whisk eggs with salt, pepper, and garlic powder.
5. Divide butternut squash and bacon evenly among muffin cups.
6. Pour egg mixture over the top and bake for 15-20 minutes or until set.

Tip: These muffins can be stored in the fridge and reheated for a quick breakfast.

Fun Fact: Butternut squash is rich in vitamins A and C, both of which are important for a healthy immune system.

7. Cauliflower Breakfast Rice

Prep Time: 20 minutes

Ingredients:

- 1 head of cauliflower, riced
- 1 tbsp coconut oil
- 1 small onion, diced
- 1 bell pepper, diced
- 2 cloves garlic, minced
- 1/2 tsp turmeric
- 1/2 tsp sea salt
- 1/4 tsp black pepper (optional for strict AIP)
- Fresh cilantro for garnish

Instructions:

1. Heat coconut oil in a skillet over medium heat.
2. Add onion, bell pepper, and garlic, cooking until the onion is translucent.
3. Stir in cauliflower rice, turmeric, salt, and pepper.
4. Cook until cauliflower is tender, about 5-7 minutes.
5. Garnish with fresh cilantro and serve.

Tip: Add cooked ground meat for extra protein.

Fun Fact: Turmeric is a potent anti-inflammatory spice that can help reduce inflammation in the body.

8. Banana-Berry Smoothie

Prep Time: 5 minutes

Ingredients:

- 1 ripe banana
- 1/2 cup mixed berries
- 1/2 cup coconut milk
- 1 tbsp collagen powder (optional)
- 1 tsp honey (optional)

Instructions:

1. Combine all ingredients in a blender and blend until smooth.
2. Pour into a glass and enjoy immediately.

Tip: Freeze the banana and berries for a thicker smoothie.

Fun Fact: Berries are high in antioxidants, which help protect your cells from damage.

9. Sausage and Spinach Breakfast Skillet

Prep Time: 20 minutes

Ingredients:

- 1 lb AIP-friendly sausage
- 2 cups fresh spinach
- 1 small onion, diced
- 1 tbsp coconut oil
- Sea salt and black pepper (optional for strict AIP) to taste

Instructions:

1. Heat coconut oil in a skillet over medium heat.
2. Add sausage and cook until browned.
3. Add onion and cook until translucent.
4. Stir in spinach and cook until wilted.
5. Season with salt and pepper to taste and serve.

Tip: Use a variety of leafy greens for different nutrients and flavors.

Fun Fact: Spinach is rich in iron, which is essential for healthy blood cells.

10. Coconut Flour Porridge

Prep Time: 10 minutes

Ingredients:

- 1/4 cup coconut flour
- 1 cup coconut milk
- 1/4 tsp sea salt
- 1 tsp honey (optional)
- Fresh fruit for topping

Instructions:

1. In a small saucepan, combine coconut flour, coconut milk, and salt.
2. Cook over medium heat, stirring constantly, until thickened.
3. Remove from heat and stir in honey if using.
4. Top with fresh fruit and serve.

Tip: Add a pinch of cinnamon for extra flavor.

Fun Fact: Coconut flour is high in fiber and has a low glycemic index, making it a great choice for blood sugar control.

11. Zucchini Fritters

Prep Time: 25 minutes

Ingredients:

- 2 medium zucchinis, grated
- 1 egg (or 1 tbsp gelatin dissolved in 2 tbsp water for egg-free)
- 1/4 cup coconut flour
- 1/4 tsp sea salt
- 1/4 tsp black pepper (optional for strict AIP)
- Coconut oil for frying

Instructions:

1. Grate zucchini and squeeze out excess moisture.
2. In a bowl, combine zucchini, egg, coconut flour, salt, and pepper.
3. Heat coconut oil in a skillet over medium heat.
4. Scoop batter into the skillet and flatten with a spatula.
5. Cook until golden brown on both sides.
6. Serve warm.

Tip: Serve with a side of avocado for added healthy fats.

Fun Fact: Zucchini is low in calories and high in vitamins C and A.

12. Berry and Chia Seed Pudding

Prep Time: 10 minutes (plus overnight chilling)

Ingredients (continued):

- 1 tsp honey (optional)
- 1/2 tsp vanilla extract (optional)
- 1/2 cup mixed berries

Instructions:

1. In a bowl, combine chia seeds, coconut milk, honey, and vanilla extract if using.
2. Stir well and let sit for 5 minutes, then stir again to prevent clumping.
3. Cover and refrigerate overnight.
4. Serve topped with mixed berries.

Tip: Prepare a few servings at once to have a quick breakfast ready for several days.

Fun Fact: Chia seeds can absorb up to 12 times their weight in liquid, forming a gel-like consistency.

13. AIP Breakfast Sausage Patties

Prep Time: 20 minutes

Ingredients:

- 1 lb ground pork or chicken
- 1 tsp sea salt
- 1/2 tsp garlic powder
- 1/2 tsp onion powder
- 1/2 tsp dried sage
- 1/2 tsp dried thyme
- 1/4 tsp ground ginger

- 1/4 tsp ground black pepper (optional for strict AIP)
- Coconut oil for frying

Instructions:

1. In a large bowl, combine ground meat and seasonings, mixing well.
2. Form into small patties.
3. Heat coconut oil in a skillet over medium heat.
4. Cook patties until browned and cooked through, about 5 minutes per side.
5. Serve hot.

Tip: Make a large batch and freeze leftovers for quick reheating.

Fun Fact: Sage has antioxidant properties and has been traditionally used to support digestion.

14. AIP-Friendly Green Smoothie

Prep Time: 5 minutes

Ingredients:

- 1 cup spinach
- 1/2 avocado
- 1/2 cucumber, chopped
- 1/2 green apple, chopped
- 1 cup coconut water
- 1 tbsp fresh lemon juice

Instructions:

1. Combine all ingredients in a blender.
2. Blend until smooth.

3. Pour into a glass and serve immediately.

Tip: Add a handful of fresh herbs like parsley or cilantro for an extra nutrient boost.

Fun Fact: Green apples contain less sugar and more fiber compared to red apples, making them a healthier choice for smoothies.

15. Carrot and Apple Breakfast Bake

Prep Time: 40 minutes

Ingredients:

- 2 large carrots, grated
- 2 apples, peeled and grated
- 1/2 cup coconut flour
- 2 eggs (or 2 tbsp gelatin dissolved in 4 tbsp water for egg-free)
- 1/4 cup coconut oil, melted
- 1/4 cup honey
- 1 tsp ground cinnamon
- 1/2 tsp sea salt

Instructions:

1. Preheat oven to 350°F (175°C) and grease a baking dish.
2. In a large bowl, combine grated carrots, grated apples, coconut flour, eggs, coconut oil, honey, cinnamon, and salt.
3. Mix well until all ingredients are evenly incorporated.
4. Spread the mixture evenly in the baking dish.
5. Bake for 25-30 minutes, or until golden brown and set.

6. Let cool slightly before serving.

Tip: Store leftovers in the refrigerator and reheat for a quick breakfast.

Fun Fact: Carrots are rich in beta-carotene, which supports good vision and immune function.

LUNCH

1. Lemon Herb Chicken Salad

Prep Time: 30 minutes

Ingredients:

- 2 boneless, skinless chicken breasts
- 1 lemon, juiced
- 1/4 cup olive oil
- 1 tbsp fresh thyme, chopped
- 1 tbsp fresh rosemary, chopped
- 4 cups mixed greens
- 1 cucumber, sliced
- 1/2 red onion, thinly sliced
- Sea salt and black pepper (optional for strict AIP) to taste

Instructions:

1. Marinate chicken in lemon juice, olive oil, thyme, rosemary, salt, and pepper for at least 15 minutes.
2. Grill or bake chicken until fully cooked, then let it rest before slicing.
3. Arrange mixed greens, cucumber, and red onion on a plate.
4. Top with sliced chicken and drizzle with additional olive oil and lemon juice.

Tip: Marinate the chicken overnight for more intense flavors.

Fun Fact: Thyme and rosemary are known for their antimicrobial properties, which can help support a healthy immune system.

2. Shrimp and Avocado Salad

Prep Time: 20 minutes

Ingredients:

- 1 lb shrimp, peeled and deveined
- 2 avocados, diced
- 1 cup cherry tomatoes, halved
- 1/4 cup red onion, diced
- 1 lime, juiced
- 2 tbsp olive oil
- Sea salt and black pepper (optional for strict AIP) to taste

Instructions:

1. Sauté shrimp in a pan with olive oil until pink and cooked through.
2. In a bowl, combine avocado, cherry tomatoes, red onion, and cooked shrimp.
3. Drizzle with lime juice and season with salt and pepper.
4. Toss gently and serve.

Tip: Use pre-cooked shrimp to save time.

Fun Fact: Avocados are rich in monounsaturated fats, which are heart-healthy and help to absorb fat-soluble vitamins.

3. Turkey and Zucchini Meatballs

Prep Time: 35 minutes

Ingredients:

- 1 lb ground turkey
- 1 medium zucchini, grated
- 1 egg (or 1 tbsp gelatin dissolved in 2 tbsp water for egg-free)
- 1/4 cup coconut flour
- 1/2 tsp garlic powder
- 1/2 tsp onion powder
- 1/2 tsp sea salt
- 1/4 tsp black pepper (optional for strict AIP)
- Coconut oil for baking

Instructions:

1. Preheat oven to 375°F (190°C) and grease a baking sheet with coconut oil.
2. In a bowl, combine all ingredients and mix well.
3. Form into small meatballs and place on the baking sheet.
4. Bake for 25-30 minutes, or until cooked through and golden brown.

Tip: Serve with a side of marinara sauce made from tomatoes, garlic, and olive oil.

Fun Fact: Zucchini adds moisture to the meatballs and is a great source of vitamin C.

4. Sweet Potato and Kale Hash

Prep Time: 25 minutes

Ingredients:

- 2 medium sweet potatoes, peeled and diced
- 2 cups kale, chopped
- 1 small onion, diced
- 2 tbsp coconut oil

- 1 tsp sea salt
- 1/4 tsp black pepper (optional for strict AIP)

Instructions:

1. Heat coconut oil in a large skillet over medium heat.
2. Add diced sweet potatoes and cook until they start to soften, about 10 minutes.
3. Add onion and kale, cooking until the onion is translucent and the kale is wilted.
4. Season with salt and pepper and serve hot.

Tip: Add cooked ground meat for extra protein.

Fun Fact: Kale is one of the most nutrient-dense foods, packed with vitamins A, K, and C.

5. Cauliflower Fried Rice

Prep Time: 20 minutes

Ingredients:

- 1 head of cauliflower, riced
- 1 cup peas and carrots mix (use fresh or frozen)
- 2 eggs (or 2 tbsp gelatin dissolved in 4 tbsp water for egg-free)
- 1 small onion, diced
- 2 cloves garlic, minced
- 2 tbsp coconut aminos
- 1 tbsp coconut oil
- Sea salt to taste

Instructions:

1. Heat coconut oil in a large skillet over medium heat.
2. Add onion and garlic, cooking until the onion is translucent.
3. Stir in peas and carrots and cook for a few minutes.
4. Add cauliflower rice and coconut aminos, stirring well.
5. Create a well in the center of the skillet and pour in the beaten eggs, scrambling them until cooked.
6. Mix everything together and season with salt.

Tip: Use a food processor to quickly rice the cauliflower.

Fun Fact: Cauliflower is a versatile low-carb substitute for rice, providing vitamins C and K.

6. Baked Salmon with Dill Sauce

Prep Time: 30 minutes

Ingredients:

- 4 salmon fillets
- 1 lemon, sliced
- 1/4 cup fresh dill, chopped
- 1/2 cup coconut yogurt
- 1 tbsp lemon juice
- Sea salt and black pepper (optional for strict AIP) to taste

Instructions:

1. Preheat oven to 375°F (190°C).

2. Place salmon fillets on a baking sheet and top with lemon slices.
3. Bake for 20-25 minutes or until salmon is cooked through.
4. In a small bowl, mix coconut yogurt, lemon juice, dill, salt, and pepper.
5. Serve salmon with a dollop of dill sauce.

Tip: Pair with roasted vegetables for a complete meal.

Fun Fact: Salmon is rich in omega-3 fatty acids, which are beneficial for heart and brain health.

7. Chicken and Vegetable Stir-Fry

Prep Time: 25 minutes

Ingredients:

- 2 chicken breasts, sliced thinly
- 1 red bell pepper, sliced
- 1 yellow bell pepper, sliced
- 1 zucchini, sliced
- 1 small onion, sliced
- 2 cloves garlic, minced
- 2 tbsp coconut aminos
- 1 tbsp coconut oil
- Sea salt and black pepper (optional for strict AIP) to taste

Instructions:

1. Heat coconut oil in a large skillet over medium-high heat.
2. Add chicken slices and cook until browned and cooked through.

3. Remove chicken from skillet and set aside.
4. Add bell peppers, zucchini, onion, and garlic to the skillet, cooking until tender.
5. Return chicken to the skillet and stir in coconut aminos, salt, and pepper.
6. Serve hot.

Tip: Use a variety of colorful vegetables for added nutrients and flavors.

Fun Fact: Bell peppers are high in vitamin C, which supports the immune system.

8. Beef and Broccoli Stir-Fry

Prep Time: 20 minutes

Ingredients:

- 1 lb beef sirloin, thinly sliced
- 2 cups broccoli florets
- 1 small onion, sliced
- 2 cloves garlic, minced
- 2 tbsp coconut aminos
- 1 tbsp coconut oil
- Sea salt and black pepper (optional for strict AIP) to taste

Instructions:

1. Heat coconut oil in a large skillet over medium-high heat.
2. Add beef slices and cook until browned.
3. Remove beef from skillet and set aside.
4. Add broccoli, onion, and garlic to the skillet, cooking until tender.

5. Return beef to the skillet and stir in coconut aminos, salt, and pepper.
6. Serve hot.

Tip: Use pre-cut broccoli to save time.

Fun Fact: Broccoli is a cruciferous vegetable that contains compounds beneficial for detoxification.

9. Stuffed Bell Peppers

Prep Time: 45 minutes

Ingredients:

- 4 bell peppers, tops removed and seeded
- 1 lb ground beef or turkey
- 1 small onion, diced
- 1 cup cauliflower rice
- 1 cup tomato sauce (AIP-friendly)
- 2 cloves garlic, minced
- 1 tsp sea salt
- 1/4 tsp black pepper (optional for strict AIP)

Instructions:

1. Preheat oven to 375°F (190°C).
2. In a skillet, cook ground meat with onion and garlic until browned.
3. Stir in cauliflower rice, tomato sauce, salt, and pepper.
4. Stuff bell peppers with the meat mixture and place in a baking dish.
5. Cover with foil and bake for 30-35 minutes.
6. Remove foil and bake for an additional 10 minutes.

Tip: Use different colored bell peppers for a vibrant presentation.

Fun Fact: Bell peppers contain carotenoids, which are beneficial for eye health.

10. AIP Tuna Salad

Prep Time: 15 minutes

Ingredients:

- 2 cans tuna, drained
- 1/2 cup diced celery
- 1/4 cup diced red onion
- 1/4 cup diced pickles (AIP-friendly)
- 1/4 cup coconut yogurt
- 1 tbsp lemon juice
- Sea salt and black pepper (optional for strict AIP) to taste

Instructions:

1. In a bowl, combine tuna, celery, red onion, and pickles.
2. Stir in coconut yogurt, lemon juice, salt, and pepper.
3. Serve on a bed of lettuce or in a lettuce wrap.

Tip: Chill the salad in the refrigerator for an hour to let the flavors meld together.

Fun Fact: Tuna is a good source of lean protein and provides essential omega-3 fatty acids.

11. Spaghetti Squash with AIP Meat Sauce

Prep Time: 40 minutes

Ingredients:

- 1 medium spaghetti squash
- 1 lb ground beef or turkey
- 1 cup AIP-friendly tomato sauce
- 1 small onion, diced
- 2 cloves garlic, minced
- 1 tsp dried oregano
- 1 tsp dried basil
- Sea salt and black pepper (optional for strict AIP) to taste

Instructions:

1. Preheat oven to 400°F (200°C). Cut spaghetti squash in half lengthwise and remove seeds.
2. Place squash cut-side down on a baking sheet and bake for 35-40 minutes, or until tender.
3. While squash is baking, cook ground meat with onion and garlic in a skillet until browned.
4. Stir in tomato sauce, oregano, basil, salt, and pepper. Simmer for 10 minutes.
5. Scrape the flesh of the cooked squash with a fork to create "noodles."
6. Top spaghetti squash with meat sauce and serve.

Tip: For added flavor, roast the squash with a drizzle of olive oil.

Fun Fact: Spaghetti squash is a low-carb alternative to traditional pasta and provides a good source of fiber.

12. AIP Chicken Soup

Prep Time: 45 minutes

Ingredients:

- 2 cups chicken broth (AIP-friendly)
- 2 cups cooked chicken, shredded
- 1 cup carrots, diced
- 1 cup celery, diced
- 1 small onion, diced
- 2 cloves garlic, minced
- 1 bay leaf
- 1 tsp dried thyme
- Sea salt and black pepper (optional for strict AIP) to taste

Instructions:

1. In a large pot, heat a splash of oil and sauté onion, garlic, carrots, and celery until soft.
2. Add chicken broth, shredded chicken, bay leaf, thyme, salt, and pepper.
3. Bring to a boil, then reduce heat and simmer for 20 minutes.
4. Remove bay leaf before serving.

Tip: For a thicker soup, blend a portion of the soup and then mix it back in.

Fun Fact: Homemade chicken soup can be soothing and is traditionally used to support immune function.

13. AIP Roasted Chicken Thighs

Prep Time: 50 minutes

Ingredients:

- 4 bone-in chicken thighs
- 2 tbsp olive oil
- 1 lemon, sliced
- 2 tsp dried rosemary
- 1 tsp dried thyme
- Sea salt and black pepper (optional for strict AIP) to taste

Instructions:

1. Preheat oven to 400°F (200°C).
2. Rub chicken thighs with olive oil, rosemary, thyme, salt, and pepper.
3. Place chicken on a baking sheet and top with lemon slices.
4. Roast for 35-40 minutes, or until the chicken reaches an internal temperature of 165°F (74°C).

Tip: Serve with a side of roasted vegetables for a complete meal.

Fun Fact: Rosemary and thyme are aromatic herbs that not only enhance flavor but also have anti-inflammatory properties.

14. AIP Stuffed Acorn Squash

Prep Time: 40 minutes

Ingredients:

- 2 acorn squashes, halved and seeded
- 1/2 lb ground turkey or beef
- 1 small onion, diced
- 1/2 cup cooked quinoa (optional for non-strict AIP)

- 1 tsp dried sage
- 1/2 tsp sea salt
- 1/4 tsp black pepper (optional for strict AIP)

Instructions:

1. Preheat oven to 375°F (190°C).
2. Roast acorn squash halves, cut side down, on a baking sheet for 30 minutes.
3. Meanwhile, cook ground meat with onion, sage, salt, and pepper until browned.
4. Remove squash from oven and turn cut side up.
5. Stuff each squash half with the meat mixture and return to the oven for an additional 10 minutes.

Tip: If using quinoa, mix it into the meat filling for added texture.

Fun Fact: Acorn squash is rich in antioxidants and vitamins, including A and C.

15. AIP Beef and Sweet Potato Stew

Prep Time: 50 minutes

Ingredients:

- 1 lb beef stew meat
- 2 large sweet potatoes, peeled and diced
- 2 cups beef broth (AIP-friendly)
- 1 cup carrots, sliced
- 1 small onion, diced
- 2 cloves garlic, minced
- 1 tsp dried thyme

- Sea salt and black pepper (optional for strict AIP) to taste

Instructions:

1. In a large pot, brown beef stew meat with a splash of oil.
2. Add onion, garlic, carrots, and sweet potatoes, cooking until softened.
3. Stir in beef broth, thyme, salt, and pepper.
4. Bring to a boil, then reduce heat and simmer for 30-40 minutes, or until beef is tender.

Tip: Allow the stew to cool before storing in the refrigerator; flavors improve overnight.

Fun Fact: Sweet potatoes are an excellent source of beta-carotene and dietary fiber.

16. AIP Turkey Lettuce Wraps

Prep Time: 20 minutes

Ingredients:

- 1 lb ground turkey
- 1/2 cup diced bell peppers
- 1/2 cup diced onions
- 2 cloves garlic, minced
- 1 tbsp coconut aminos
- 1 tsp dried ginger
- Large lettuce leaves (for wrapping)

Instructions:

1. Cook ground turkey in a skillet until browned.

2. Add bell peppers, onions, and garlic, cooking until vegetables are tender.
3. Stir in coconut aminos and ginger.
4. Spoon turkey mixture onto lettuce leaves and wrap.

Tip: Use a variety of colorful bell peppers for added nutrients.

Fun Fact: Lettuce wraps are a great low-carb alternative to tortillas or bread.

17. AIP Mediterranean Chicken

Prep Time: 30 minutes

Ingredients:

- 4 boneless, skinless chicken thighs
- 1/2 cup black olives, sliced
- 1/2 cup sun-dried tomatoes, chopped
- 1/4 cup fresh basil, chopped
- 2 tbsp olive oil
- Sea salt and black pepper (optional for strict AIP) to taste

Instructions:

1. Preheat oven to 375°F (190°C).
2. Rub chicken thighs with olive oil, salt, and pepper.
3. Place chicken in a baking dish and top with olives, sun-dried tomatoes, and basil.
4. Bake for 25-30 minutes, or until chicken is cooked through.

Tip: Serve with a side of roasted vegetables or a fresh green salad.

Fun Fact: Sun-dried tomatoes are concentrated in antioxidants and vitamins, adding a rich flavor to dishes.

18. AIP Spaghetti Squash with Pesto

Prep Time: 30 minutes

Ingredients:

- 1 medium spaghetti squash
- 1/2 cup fresh basil leaves
- 1/4 cup pine nuts (or seeds for AIP)
- 1/4 cup olive oil
- 1 clove garlic
- Sea salt to taste

Instructions:

1. Preheat oven to 400°F (200°C). Cut spaghetti squash in half and remove seeds.
2. Roast squash cut-side down on a baking sheet for 35-40 minutes.
3. In a food processor, blend basil, pine nuts, olive oil, and garlic until smooth.
4. Scrape the flesh of the squash into "noodles" and toss with pesto.

Tip: Prepare the pesto in advance and store it in the refrigerator for up to a week.

Fun Fact: Basil has anti-inflammatory properties and is rich in antioxidants.

19. AIP Chicken and Vegetable Skewers

Prep Time: 25 minutes

Ingredients:

- 1 lb chicken breast, cubed
- 1 red bell pepper, cut into chunks
- 1 zucchini, sliced
- 1/2 red onion, cut into chunks
- 2 tbsp olive oil
- 1 tsp dried oregano
- Sea salt and black pepper (optional for strict AIP) to taste

Instructions:

1. Preheat grill to medium-high heat.
2. Thread chicken and vegetables onto skewers.
3. Brush with olive oil and season with oregano, salt, and pepper.
4. Grill for 10-15 minutes, turning occasionally, until chicken is cooked through.

Tip: Soak wooden skewers in water before grilling to prevent burning.

Fun Fact: Grilling adds a smoky flavor to food without the need for additional fats.

20. AIP Chicken and Apple Salad

Prep Time: 15 minutes

Ingredients:

- 2 cups cooked chicken, shredded

- 1 large apple, diced
- 1/4 cup celery, diced
- 1/4 cup walnuts (optional for AIP)
- 1/4 cup coconut yogurt
- 1 tbsp apple cider vinegar
- Sea salt and black pepper (optional for strict AIP) to taste

Instructions:

1. In a bowl, combine chicken, apple, celery, and walnuts.
2. Stir in coconut yogurt, apple cider vinegar, salt, and pepper.
3. Mix well and serve on

DINNER

1. AIP Herb-Roasted Chicken

Prep Time: 1 hour

Ingredients:

- 1 whole chicken (about 4 lbs)
- 2 tbsp olive oil
- 2 tbsp fresh rosemary, chopped
- 2 tbsp fresh thyme, chopped
- 1 lemon, quartered
- Sea salt and black pepper (optional for strict AIP)

Instructions:

1. Preheat oven to 375°F (190°C).
2. Rub the chicken with olive oil, rosemary, thyme, salt, and pepper.
3. Place lemon quarters inside the cavity.
4. Roast for 1 hour or until the internal temperature reaches 165°F (74°C).

Tip: Let the chicken rest for 10 minutes before carving to retain juices.

Fun Fact: Rosemary is known to have antioxidant and anti-inflammatory properties.

2. Stuffed Acorn Squash with Ground Turkey

Prep Time: 50 minutes

Ingredients:

- 2 acorn squashes, halved and seeded
- 1 lb ground turkey
- 1 small onion, diced
- 1/2 cup chopped apple
- 1 tsp dried sage
- Sea salt and black pepper (optional for strict AIP)

Instructions:

1. Preheat oven to 375°F (190°C).
2. Roast squash halves cut-side down for 30 minutes.
3. Cook ground turkey with onion, apple, sage, salt, and pepper.
4. Stuff roasted squash with the turkey mixture and bake for an additional 10 minutes.

Tip: Use a fork to check if the squash is tender.

Fun Fact: Acorn squash is rich in vitamins A and C.

3. AIP Beef and Sweet Potato Chili

Prep Time: 1 hour

Ingredients:

- 1 lb ground beef
- 2 large sweet potatoes, peeled and diced
- 1 cup diced tomatoes (AIP-friendly)
- 1 cup beef broth (AIP-friendly)
- 1 small onion, diced
- 2 cloves garlic, minced
- 1 tsp ground cumin
- Sea salt to taste

Instructions:

1. Cook ground beef with onion and garlic until browned.
2. Add sweet potatoes, tomatoes, beef broth, cumin, and salt.
3. Simmer for 45 minutes, or until sweet potatoes are tender.

Tip: For a thicker chili, mash some of the sweet potatoes in the pot.

Fun Fact: Sweet potatoes are high in fiber, which supports digestive health.

4. Baked Cod with Lemon and Dill

Prep Time: 25 minutes

Ingredients:

- 4 cod fillets
- 1 lemon, sliced
- 2 tbsp fresh dill, chopped
- 2 tbsp olive oil
- Sea salt and black pepper (optional for strict AIP)

Instructions:

1. Preheat oven to 400°F (200°C).
2. Place cod fillets on a baking sheet, drizzle with olive oil, and top with lemon slices and dill.
3. Bake for 15-20 minutes, or until fish flakes easily with a fork.

Tip: Serve with steamed vegetables or a side salad.

Fun Fact: Cod is a good source of lean protein and vitamin B12.

5. AIP Coconut Curry Chicken

Prep Time: 30 minutes

Ingredients:

- 1 lb chicken thighs, cubed
- 1 can coconut milk
- 2 tbsp curry powder (AIP-friendly)
- 1 cup diced butternut squash
- 1 cup spinach
- Sea salt to taste

Instructions:

1. In a pot, cook chicken until browned.
2. Add curry powder, coconut milk, and butternut squash.
3. Simmer for 20 minutes, or until squash is tender.
4. Stir in spinach until wilted.

Tip: Adjust the amount of curry powder to control the spice level.

Fun Fact: Coconut milk provides a creamy texture and is a good source of healthy fats.

6. AIP Grilled Salmon with Avocado Salsa

Prep Time: 20 minutes

Ingredients:

- 4 salmon fillets
- 1 avocado, diced
- 1 tomato, diced
- 1/4 cup red onion, diced
- 1 lime, juiced
- Sea salt to taste

Instructions:

1. Preheat grill to medium-high heat.
2. Season salmon fillets with salt and grill for 4-5 minutes per side.
3. In a bowl, combine avocado, tomato, red onion, and lime juice.
4. Serve salmon topped with avocado salsa.

Tip: Use a fish basket to prevent the salmon from sticking to the grill.

Fun Fact: Avocado salsa adds healthy fats and enhances the flavor of grilled fish.

7. AIP Pork Tenderloin with Roasted Apples

Prep Time: 40 minutes

Ingredients:

- 1 lb pork tenderloin
- 2 apples, sliced
- 2 tbsp olive oil
- 1 tsp dried thyme
- Sea salt and black pepper (optional for strict AIP)

Instructions:

1. Preheat oven to 400°F (200°C).
2. Rub pork tenderloin with olive oil, thyme, salt, and pepper.
3. Place tenderloin in a baking dish and surround with apple slices.
4. Roast for 25-30 minutes, or until pork reaches an internal temperature of 145°F (63°C).

Tip: Let the pork rest for 10 minutes before slicing.

Fun Fact: Apples add a natural sweetness to savory dishes.

8. AIP Chicken and Vegetable Skillet

Prep Time: 30 minutes

Ingredients:

- 2 chicken breasts, diced
- 1 cup broccoli florets
- 1 red bell pepper, diced
- 1 small zucchini, sliced
- 2 tbsp olive oil
- 1 tsp dried oregano
- Sea salt and black pepper (optional for strict AIP)

Instructions:

1. Heat olive oil in a skillet over medium heat.
2. Cook chicken until browned and cooked through.
3. Add broccoli, bell pepper, and zucchini, cooking until vegetables are tender.
4. Season with oregano, salt, and pepper.

Tip: Use a lid to help steam the vegetables for quicker cooking.

Fun Fact: Skillet meals are a great way to cook everything in one pan, reducing cleanup time.

9. AIP Stuffed Bell Peppers

Prep Time: 45 minutes

Ingredients:

- 4 bell peppers, tops removed and seeded
- 1 lb ground beef
- 1/2 cup cauliflower rice
- 1/2 cup tomato sauce (AIP-friendly)
- 1 tsp dried basil
- Sea salt to taste

Instructions:

1. Preheat oven to 375°F (190°C).
2. Cook ground beef with cauliflower rice, tomato sauce, basil, and salt.
3. Stuff bell peppers with the beef mixture.
4. Bake for 30-35 minutes.

Tip: Use different colored bell peppers for visual appeal.

Fun Fact: Cauliflower rice adds a low-carb alternative to traditional rice in stuffed peppers.

10. AIP Lemon Garlic Shrimp

Prep Time: 15 minutes

Ingredients:

- 1 lb shrimp, peeled and deveined
- 3 cloves garlic, minced
- 1 lemon, juiced
- 2 tbsp olive oil
- Sea salt and black pepper (optional for strict AIP)

Instructions:

1. Heat olive oil in a pan over medium heat.
2. Add garlic and cook until fragrant.
3. Add shrimp and cook until pink and opaque, about 3-4 minutes per side.
4. Stir in lemon juice and season with salt and pepper.

Tip: Serve with a side of steamed vegetables or over a bed of lettuce.

Fun Fact: Shrimp is high in protein and provides essential nutrients like selenium.

11. AIP Chicken Thighs with Roasted Brussels Sprouts

Prep Time: 40 minutes

Ingredients:

- 4 chicken thighs
- 2 cups Brussels sprouts, halved
- 2 tbsp olive oil
- 1 tsp dried thyme
- Sea salt to taste

Instructions:

1. Preheat oven to 400°F (200°C).
2. Rub chicken thighs with olive oil, thyme, and salt.
3. Place on a baking sheet and surround with Brussels sprouts.
4. Roast for 30-35 minutes, or until chicken reaches an internal temperature of 165°F (74°C).

Tip: Toss Brussels sprouts with a bit of olive oil and sea salt before roasting.

Fun Fact: Brussels sprouts are high in fiber and vitamins C and K.

12. AIP Balsamic Glazed Chicken

Prep Time: 30 minutes

Ingredients:

- 4 chicken breasts
- 1/4 cup balsamic vinegar
- 2 tbsp olive oil
- 1 tsp dried rosemary
- Sea salt and black pepper (optional for strict AIP)

Instructions:

1. Preheat oven to 375°F (190°C).
2. Rub chicken breasts with olive oil, rosemary, salt, and pepper.
3. Place in a baking dish and drizzle with balsamic vinegar.

4. Bake for 25-30 minutes.

Tip: Allow the chicken to rest before slicing to retain juices.

Fun Fact: Balsamic vinegar adds a tangy sweetness that enhances the flavor of chicken.

13. AIP Butternut Squash Soup

Prep Time: 45 minutes

Ingredients:

- 1 small onion, diced
- 2 cloves garlic, minced
- 4 cups chicken broth (AIP-friendly)
- 2 tbsp olive oil
- 1 tsp dried sage
- Sea salt to taste

Instructions:

1. Preheat oven to 400°F (200°C). Toss butternut squash with olive oil and salt, then roast for 25-30 minutes until tender.
2. In a pot, sauté onion and garlic until soft.
3. Add roasted squash and chicken broth. Simmer for 10 minutes.
4. Blend the soup until smooth using an immersion blender or stand blender.
5. Stir in sage and adjust seasoning if needed.

Tip: Garnish with a swirl of coconut cream for added richness.

Fun Fact: Butternut squash is rich in vitamins A and C, and its natural sweetness enhances soups.

14. AIP Zucchini Noodles with Meatballs

Prep Time: 35 minutes

Ingredients:

- 2 large zucchinis, spiralized into noodles
- 1 lb ground beef
- 1/4 cup coconut flour
- 1 egg (or egg substitute for strict AIP)
- 1 tsp dried oregano
- 1/2 tsp garlic powder
- 1 cup AIP-friendly tomato sauce

Instructions:

1. Preheat oven to 375°F (190°C).
2. Mix ground beef with coconut flour, egg, oregano, and garlic powder. Form into meatballs and place on a baking sheet.
3. Bake meatballs for 20-25 minutes.
4. Heat zucchini noodles in a pan until just tender.
5. Serve meatballs over zucchini noodles with tomato sauce.

Tip: You can use a spiralizer or a julienne peeler to create zucchini noodles.

Fun Fact: Zucchini noodles are a low-carb alternative to traditional pasta.

15. AIP Miso Glazed Chicken

Prep Time: 30 minutes

Ingredients:

- 4 chicken thighs
- 2 tbsp coconut aminos
- 1 tbsp AIP-friendly miso paste (or coconut aminos for stricter AIP)
- 2 tbsp olive oil
- Sea salt to taste

Instructions:

1. Preheat oven to 375°F (190°C).
2. Mix coconut aminos and miso paste to make the glaze.
3. Brush chicken thighs with the glaze and place in a baking dish.
4. Bake for 25-30 minutes, or until chicken reaches 165°F (74°C).

Tip: Brush the chicken with additional glaze halfway through baking for more flavor.

Fun Fact: Coconut aminos is a soy sauce substitute made from fermented coconut sap and is often used in AIP recipes.

16. AIP Cauliflower and Chicken Curry

Prep Time: 35 minutes

Ingredients:

- 1 lb chicken breasts, cubed
- 1 head cauliflower, cut into florets
- 1 can coconut milk
- 2 tbsp curry powder (AIP-friendly)
- 1 small onion, diced

- 2 cloves garlic, minced
- Sea salt to taste

Instructions:

1. Sauté onion and garlic in a pan until soft.
2. Add chicken and cook until browned.
3. Stir in curry powder, coconut milk, and cauliflower.
4. Simmer for 20 minutes or until cauliflower is tender.

Tip: Serve with a side of steamed greens or cauliflower rice.

Fun Fact: Curry powder can add depth and warmth to dishes, and coconut milk provides a creamy base.

17. AIP Pork and Apple Skillet

Prep Time: 30 minutes

Ingredients:

- 1 lb pork loin, sliced
- 2 apples, sliced
- 1 tbsp olive oil
- 1 tsp dried sage
- Sea salt and black pepper (optional for strict AIP)

Instructions:

1. Heat olive oil in a skillet over medium heat.
2. Cook pork slices until browned on both sides.
3. Add apple slices and sage, cooking until apples are tender and pork is cooked through.

Tip: Use a lid to help the apples cook faster and to keep the pork moist.

Fun Fact: Apples add natural sweetness and enhance the flavor of savory dishes.

18. AIP Turkey Meatloaf

Prep Time: 50 minutes

Ingredients:

- 1 lb ground turkey
- 1/2 cup grated carrot
- 1/2 cup finely chopped onion
- 2 cloves garlic, minced
- 1/4 cup coconut flour
- 1 egg (or egg substitute for strict AIP)
- 1 tsp dried thyme
- Sea salt to taste

Instructions:

1. Preheat oven to 375°F (190°C).
2. Mix all ingredients in a bowl and form into a loaf shape.
3. Place in a baking dish and bake for 35-40 minutes.

Tip: Let the meatloaf rest for 10 minutes before slicing.

Fun Fact: Coconut flour helps to bind the meatloaf and adds a subtle flavor.

19. AIP Baked Eggplant with Tomato Sauce

Prep Time: 45 minutes

Ingredients:

- 2 large eggplants, sliced
- 1 cup AIP-friendly tomato sauce
- 2 tbsp olive oil
- 1 tsp dried basil
- Sea salt to taste

Instructions:

1. Preheat oven to 375°F (190°C).
2. Brush eggplant slices with olive oil and bake for 20 minutes.
3. Top eggplant slices with tomato sauce and basil, then bake for an additional 15 minutes.

Tip: Sprinkle with fresh basil before serving for extra flavor.

Fun Fact: Eggplant is rich in antioxidants and adds a meaty texture to dishes.

20. AIP Lemon Herb Baked Salmon

Prep Time: 30 minutes

Ingredients:

- 4 salmon fillets
- 1 lemon, thinly sliced
- 2 tbsp fresh parsley, chopped
- 2 tbsp olive oil
- Sea salt and black pepper (optional for strict AIP)

Instructions:

1. Preheat oven to 400°F (200°C).
2. Place salmon fillets on a baking sheet and drizzle with olive oil.
3. Top with lemon slices and parsley.
4. Bake for 15-20 minutes, or until salmon flakes easily with a fork.

Tip: Use parchment paper on the baking sheet for easier cleanup.

Fun Fact: Salmon is an excellent source of omega-3 fatty acids and provides a healthy protein option for dinner.

SNACKS AND DESSERT

1. AIP Apple Cinnamon Chips

Prep Time: 2 hours

Ingredients:

- 2 large apples, thinly sliced
- 1 tsp ground cinnamon
- 1 tbsp lemon juice

Instructions:

1. Preheat oven to 200°F (95°C). Line a baking sheet with parchment paper.
2. Toss apple slices with lemon juice and cinnamon.
3. Arrange slices in a single layer on the baking sheet.
4. Bake for 1.5-2 hours, or until crisp, turning halfway through.

Tip: Use a mandoline for even slicing.

Fun Fact: Apples are high in fiber and antioxidants.

2. AIP Coconut Macaroons

Prep Time: 25 minutes

Ingredients:

- 2 cups shredded unsweetened coconut
- 1/2 cup coconut milk
- 1/4 cup honey
- 1/2 tsp vanilla extract (optional)

Instructions:

1. Preheat oven to 350°F (175°C). Line a baking sheet with parchment paper.
2. Mix coconut, coconut milk, honey, and vanilla extract until well combined.
3. Drop spoonfuls of the mixture onto the baking sheet.
4. Bake for 15-20 minutes, or until edges are golden brown.

Tip: Let macaroons cool completely before removing from the baking sheet.

Fun Fact: Coconut is rich in healthy fats and provides a natural sweetness.

3. AIP Chocolate Avocado Pudding

Prep Time: 10 minutes

Ingredients:

- 2 ripe avocados
- 1/4 cup raw cacao powder
- 1/4 cup honey
- 1 tsp vanilla extract (optional)
- A pinch of sea salt

Instructions:

1. Blend all ingredients in a food processor until smooth.
2. Chill in the refrigerator for at least 30 minutes before serving.

Tip: Adjust sweetness with more honey if desired.

Fun Fact: Avocados are packed with healthy fats and make a creamy base for desserts.

4. AIP Banana Coconut Energy Bites

Prep Time: 15 minutes

Ingredients:

- 1 ripe banana, mashed
- 1 cup shredded unsweetened coconut
- 1/4 cup almond butter (or another AIP-compliant nut butter)
- 1/2 tsp ground cinnamon

Instructions:

1. Mix all ingredients in a bowl until well combined.
2. Form into small balls and place on a plate.
3. Refrigerate for 1 hour before serving.

Tip: Store energy bites in the refrigerator for up to a week.

Fun Fact: Bananas add natural sweetness and are a good source of potassium.

5. AIP Chia Seed Pudding

Prep Time: 10 minutes (plus 2 hours chilling)

Ingredients:

- 1/4 cup chia seeds
- 1 cup coconut milk
- 2 tbsp honey

- 1/2 tsp vanilla extract (optional)

Instructions:

1. Mix chia seeds, coconut milk, honey, and vanilla extract in a bowl.
2. Let sit for 10 minutes, then stir again.
3. Cover and refrigerate for at least 2 hours, or until thickened.

Tip: Top with fresh berries or sliced fruit before serving.

Fun Fact: Chia seeds are high in fiber and omega-3 fatty acids.

6. AIP Baked Plantain Chips

Prep Time: 30 minutes

Ingredients:

- 2 green plantains, peeled and thinly sliced
- 2 tbsp coconut oil
- Sea salt to taste

Instructions:

1. Preheat oven to 350°F (175°C). Line a baking sheet with parchment paper.
2. Toss plantain slices with melted coconut oil and sea salt.
3. Arrange slices in a single layer on the baking sheet.
4. Bake for 15-20 minutes, flipping halfway through, until crispy.

Tip: Keep an eye on the chips to prevent burning.

Fun Fact: Plantains are rich in potassium and fiber.

7. AIP Mango Coconut Sorbet

Prep Time: 15 minutes (plus 2 hours freezing)

Ingredients:

- 2 ripe mangos, peeled and diced
- 1 cup coconut milk
- 1/4 cup honey

Instructions:

1. Blend mangos, coconut milk, and honey until smooth.
2. Pour mixture into a freezer-safe container and freeze for at least 2 hours.
3. Let sit at room temperature for 10 minutes before serving.

Tip: Stir the sorbet every 30 minutes during freezing for a smoother texture.

Fun Fact: Mangoes are high in vitamin C and add a tropical flavor to desserts.

8. AIP Pumpkin Spice Smoothie

Prep Time: 5 minutes

Ingredients:

- 1 cup canned pumpkin
- 1 cup coconut milk

- 1 tbsp honey
- 1/2 tsp pumpkin pie spice
- A pinch of sea salt

Instructions:

1. Blend all ingredients until smooth.
2. Serve immediately or chill in the refrigerator.

Tip: Adjust sweetness with more honey if desired.

Fun Fact: Pumpkin is a good source of vitamins A and C, as well as fiber.

9. AIP Pear and Berry Compote

Prep Time: 20 minutes

Ingredients:

- 2 ripe pears, peeled and diced
- 1 cup mixed berries (fresh or frozen)
- 1/4 cup honey
- 1/2 tsp vanilla extract (optional)

Instructions:

1. Combine pears, berries, honey, and vanilla extract in a saucepan.
2. Cook over medium heat until fruit is soft and mixture thickens, about 15 minutes.
3. Let cool before serving.

Tip: Serve over coconut yogurt or as a topping for AIP pancakes.

Fun Fact: Berries are rich in antioxidants and add natural sweetness to dishes.

10. AIP Coconut Almond Joy Bars

Prep Time: 30 minutes

Ingredients:

- 1 cup shredded unsweetened coconut
- 1/2 cup almond butter (or AIP-compliant nut butter)
- 1/4 cup raw cacao powder
- 1/4 cup honey
- 1/4 cup chopped almonds (optional for non-strict AIP)

Instructions:

1. Mix coconut, almond butter, cacao powder, and honey until well combined.
2. Press mixture into a lined baking dish.
3. Refrigerate for 30 minutes, then cut into bars.

Tip: Use parchment paper for easy removal from the dish.

Fun Fact: Almonds add crunch and healthy fats to these bars.